T0197671

THE OUTBREAK OF CORONAVIRUS 2020

1ST EDITION

RICHARD A. VASQUEZ

To order additional copies of this book, contact:
Xlibris
844-714-8691
www.Xlibris.com
Orders@Xlibris.com

ISBN: Softcover   978-1-6698-4497-6
         EBook   978-1-6698-4496-9

Print information available on the last page

Rev. date: 09/24/2022

CONTENTS

Preface v

Definitions vii

Introduction ix

Chapter 1 First Discovery 1

Chapter 2 The Spread of COVID-19 4

Chapter 3 Epidemic Shutdown 8

Chapter 4 Social Distancing and Remedies 15

Chapter 5 Black Lives Matter 25

Chapter 6 Conclusions 28

References 29

PREFACE

With no warning, a pandemic arose, and 2020 became a new way of understanding the unexpected. The purpose of this project is to help readers and learners know the history, development, and how to fight the coronavirus. I will give details of how COVID-19 changed everyone's way of living and thinking. As an educator, student, and public servant, I believe that this information will help provide safety and awareness of why coronavirus is a threat to all humans. This research will help readers develop information about what happened during the pandemic and what is needed to be safe for years to come.

I choose this topic because coronavirus is an ongoing problem and has affected millions of people worldwide. Just for the readers' interest and disclosure, I'm neither a physician nor have any experience in the medical field. This project is for information only and in support of the cause itself.

I will refer to the current article and events when COVID-19 started. However, COVID-19's impact put people's lives in jeopardy of seeking unanswered questions and will hide the values of how to be safe and who to trust.

Since there is no valuable information about the virus, I will give details of what has been effective to survive. I aim to enhance the readers by providing key elements of how important social distancing can be and why social distancing saves lives when near someone who had and or has COVID. It is important for readers to seek guidance from the materials that are provided.

I will also note what precautions are needed to overcome all negativity from the ongoing pandemic. Many readers will feel the daily hardships of this outbreak.

However, this research literature will define why we as educators, survivors, and learners must become aware of such virus. I will include a definition page that will provide valid information for readers.

DEFINITIONS

Acute Respiratory Distress Syndrome (ARDS): Syndrome associated with the severe coronavirus disease

Centers for Disease Control and Prevention (CDC): The leading national public health institute of the United States. It is a United States federal agency under the Department of Health and Human Services and is headquartered in Atlanta, Georgia

Chloroquine phosphate (CQ): An antimalarial drug shown to have activity against the virus that causes COVID-19 in the lab but not yet in human trials

Convalescent plasma: Blood plasma donated by persons who recovered from COVID-19 (containing natural antibodies) and is being studied as a treatment for severely ill COVID-19 patients

Coronavirus (2019-nCoV): The initial name of the novel coronavirus discovered in late 2019 in Wuhan, China, later renamed SARS-CoV-2

COVID-19 (Coronavirus Disease 2019): Official name for the disease caused by the SARS-CoV-2 (2019-nCoV) coronavirus. Informal name: Corona

Epidemic (Epi) Curve: A statistical chart used to visualize the onset and progression of a disease outbreak

Epidemiology: The study of disease and other health outcomes, their causes in a population, and how they can be controlled

Favipiravir (Avigan; T-705): Antiviral drug developed by Toyama Chemical (Fujifilm group) of Japan with activity against many RNA viruses. Being studied in China for experimental treatment of the coronavirus disease

Hydroxychloroquine (HCQ): An antimalarial drug shown to have activity against the virus that causes COVID-19 but not yet in human trials

Infection prevention and control (IPC): Strategies to prevent or limit transmission in health care settings

Influenza (Flu): is a viral infection that attacks your respiratory system, your nose, throat, and lungs. It is commonly called the flu but is not the same as stomach flu.

Outbreak: Higher than expected number of occurrences of a disease in a specific location

Social Distance: The extent to which individuals or groups are removed from or excluded from participating in one another's lives

Remdesivir (GS-5734): Antiviral drug developed by Gilead now in phase 3 clinical trials for COVID-19

Virus: An ultramicroscopic (20 to 300 nanometers in diameter), metabolically inert, infectious agent that replicates only within the cells of living hosts, mainly bacteria, plants, and animals: composed of an RNA or DNA core, a protein coat, and in more complex types, a surrounding envelope

World Health Organization (WHO): The organization that directs the international health efforts within the United Nations' system and leads with partners in global health responses

INTRODUCTION

Before the world knew anything about the coronavirus, many counted the days for adventure, longevity, family gathering, and social grouping. However, in the beginning of 2020, the outbreak of humankind for living changed forever. The outbreak of such a virus had just begun, and many were not expecting corona to be such a death-threatening dilemma. As a researcher, this perception will give notice of how fast COVID-19 has impacted many families, economy-driven businesses, and employment. The truth is the world was not prepared for such a virus.

According to Cohut (2020), dealing with the unforeseen challenges caused by the COVID-19 pandemic has taken a significant toll on people across the world. There are over 2,700,000 confirmed cases of COVID-19 across the globe. According to official reports, the largest numbers of confirmed cases are in the United States, Italy, Spain, and France.

However, even the countries where the new coronavirus has hit less aggressively are still under considerable strain. As many as 213 countries and territories have registered COVID-19 cases, and the entire world is buzzing with uncertainty and questions: How long will the pandemic last? What will people's lives look like once the pandemic is over? These are the questions that are unanswered and will still be a potential threat.

The main goal is to ensure people worldwide that we are overcomers and that we can unite for such a great cause. The pandemic has been a thorn in the bushes for many, but some can believe there is light at the end. We are fighting the boundaries that are still unanswered. However, with countries uniting, we as survivors will help those who are still victims.

1

FIRST DISCOVERY

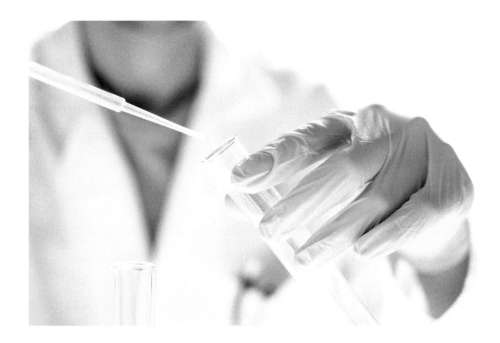

The first actions caused by human coronavirus were discovered and experimented on but were never studied with perfection. However, the breakthrough for a new virus had been uncovered. The COVID-19 name was not discovered until later after the virus was affecting humans worldwide. A common cold or flu could cause the human body to become infected by the virus, which is deadly.

The human coronavirus was first identified in the late 1960s. History states that researchers from the Common Cold Unit in Wiltshire, United Kingdom, discovered a virus that was described as virtually unrelated to any other known viruses. Thus described as the B814 could attack the human respiratory system. Therefore, we can conclude that COVID-19 came from the source of the common cold. Symptoms were sore throat, running and/or stuffy nose, which would lead some to believe that the cause of the virus was not life-threatening. Now it has been over sixty years, we are left with the unfinished business of COVID-19. The breakout still leaves a clue to the discovery, but we can't acknowledge the deadly outcome and its threat. As many remain uneducated about the history of COVID-19, some are still seeking answers.

However, according to "About COVID-19" (2020), a novel coronavirus is a new coronavirus that has not been previously identified. The virus-causing coronavirus disease 2019 (COVID-19) is not the same as the coronaviruses that commonly circulate among humans and cause mild illnesses, like the common cold. COVID-19 is caused by a coronavirus called SARS-CoV-2. Coronaviruses are a large family of viruses that are common in people and many different species of animals, including camels, cattle, cats, and bats.

On February 11, 2020, the World Health Organization announced an official name for the disease that is causing the 2019 novel coronavirus outbreak first identified in Wuhan, China. The new name of this disease is coronavirus disease 2019, abbreviated as COVID-19. In COVID-19, the CO stands for "corona," VI for "virus," and D for "disease." Formerly, this disease was referred to as "2019 novel coronavirus" or "2019-nCoV." There are many types of human coronaviruses, including some that commonly cause mild upper-respiratory tract illnesses. COVID-19 is a new disease caused by a novel (or new) coronavirus that has not previously been seen in humans.

So is it safe to say that China is the source of such a virus, COVID-19? With the marketing of the selling of animals to eat, can such source be the foundation of the actions of a common cold? These are the answers that are clueless to all that have been affected. The world has changed its image of how China conducts marketing animals for consumption. However, with the actions of China, we still know that the spread of such virus was caused by human traveling. After acknowledging these facts about COVID-19, people still did nothing to stay safe.

According to "A Timeline of COVID-19 Developments in 2020," on January 21, a Chinese scientist confirms COVID-19's human transmission. At that point, the 2019 novel coronavirus has killed four and infected more than two hundred in China before Zhong Nanshan, MD, finally confirms it can be transmitted from person to person. However, the WHO is still unsure as to the necessity of declaring a public health emergency.

On January 23, Wuhan Now Under Quarantine. In just two days, thirteen more people died and an additional three hundred became sick. China makes the unprecedented move not only to close off Wuhan and its population of eleven million but to also place a restricted access protocol on Huanggang, thirty miles to the east, and residents cannot leave without special permission. This means up to eighteen million people are under strict lockdown.

On January 31, WHO issues a global health emergency. With a worldwide death toll of more than 200 and an exponential jump to more than 9,800 cases, the WHO finally declares a public health emergency for just the sixth time. Human-to-human transmission is quickly spreading and can now be found in the United States, Germany, Japan, Vietnam, and Taiwan. On February 2, global air travel is restricted.

On February 3, the United States declares a public health emergency. The Trump administration declares a public health emergency due to the coronavirus outbreak. The announcement comes three days after WHO declared a global health emergency as more than 9,800 cases of the virus and more than 200 deaths had been confirmed worldwide.

On March 6, twenty-one passengers on a California cruise ship test positive.

Twenty-one people out of just 46 tested aboard a cruise ship carrying more than 3,500 people off the California coast test positive for COVID-19 with 19 being crew members. The ship is held at sea instead of being allowed to dock in San Francisco while testing is conducted. Since the event, 60 passengers have sued the cruise line and parent company, Carnival Corp, for gross negligence in how passenger safety was handled. This was an outlet of all possibilities for an outbreak and then media helped guild the information to support the danger of COVID-19.

Before, in 2020, the world knew nothing of such virus and imposed that it would be a short time before life went back to order. However, the timeframe of knowing when the world could overcome such pain from COVID-19 is still unanswered. We as humans blind ourselves from the secrets of the unknown. However, this secret was well known and was not life-threatening.

2

THE SPREAD OF COVID-19

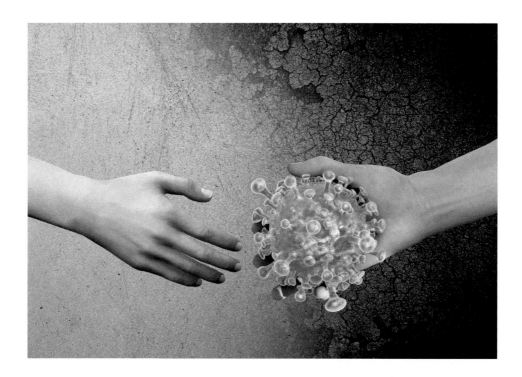

As many believed this was not a threat, most were carrying the virus without knowing its deadly outcome. Traveling was a key element that helped the process of spreading the virus. According to "About COVID-19" (2020), there is ongoing transmission of the novel coronavirus within the United States and in destinations across the world.

You may have been exposed to COVID-19 during your travels (domestic and/or international). You may feel well and not have any symptoms, but you can be contagious without symptoms and spread the virus to others. You and your travel companions (including children) pose a risk to your family, friends, and community for the fourteen days after you were exposed to the virus regardless of where you traveled or what you did during your trip. Some types of travel and activities can put you at higher risk for exposure to COVID-19. If you know that you were exposed to someone with COVID-19, postpone further travel. Even without symptoms, you can spread COVID-19 to other people on your journey. The COVID-19 virus utilized traveling as a treat to many without notice. According to "COVID-19" (2020), since December 31, 2019, and as of September 13, 2020, 28,802,775 cases of COVID-19 (in accordance with the applied case definitions and testing strategies in the affected countries) have been reported, including 920,931 deaths. The reality of a virus had just begun, and many were uncertain as to how the world could hold itself together. But with the world on the edge of its seat, the virus had its own devastation.

Cases reported worldwide: Africa: 1,347,353 cases; the five countries reporting most cases are South Africa (648,214), Egypt (100,856), Morocco (84,435), Ethiopia (63,888), and Nigeria (56,177). Asia: 8,436,613 cases; the five countries reporting the most cases are India (4,754,356), Iran (399,940), Bangladesh (336,044), Saudi Arabia (325,050), and Pakistan (301,481). America: 14,847,457 cases; the five countries reporting the most cases are United States (6,486,108), Brazil (4,315,687), Peru (722,832), Colombia (708 964), and Mexico (663 73). Europe: 4,139,193 cases; the five countries reporting the most cases are Russia (1,057,362), Spain (566,326), France (373,911), the United Kingdom (365,174), and Italy (286,297). Oceania: 31,463 cases; the five countries reporting the most cases are Australia (26,607), Guam (1,891), New Zealand (1,446), French Polynesia (891), and Papua New Guinea (510). Other: 696 cases have been reported from an international conveyance in Japan.

Deaths have been reported: Africa: 32,501 deaths; the five countries reporting the most deaths are South Africa (15427), Egypt (5,627), Algeria (1,605), Morocco (1,553), and Nigeria (1,078). Asia: 161,371 deaths; the five countries reporting the most deaths are India (78,586), Iran (23,029), Indonesia (8,650), Iraq (7,941), and Turkey (6,999). America: 512 221 deaths; the five countries reporting most deaths are the United States (193,701), Brazil (131,210), Mexico (70,604), Peru (30,593), and Colombia (22,734). Europe: 213,967 deaths; the five countries reporting most deaths are the United Kingdom (41,623), Italy (35,603), France (30,910), Spain (29,747), and Russia (18,484). Oceania: 864 deaths; the five countries reporting the most deaths are Australia (803), Guam (25), New Zealand (24), Papua New Guinea (6), and Fiji (2).

With the virus rapidly counting the days of death. Doctors, scientists, and politicians created a policy that will guarantee the safety and order against the virus. America was on the frontline along with other established countries that help identify the threat of the coronavirus disease. Some felt that the virus was going to blow over and the virus was just a common sickness.

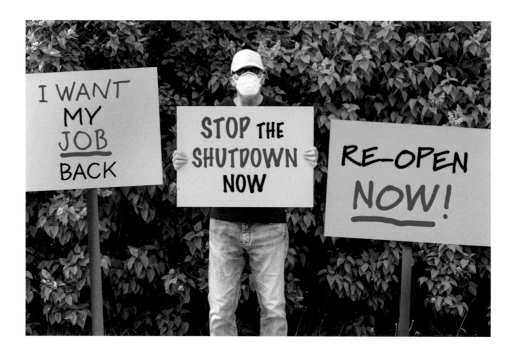

But once the spread started, many were convinced that it was a global epidemic. Thus, creating a need for the necessities-of-home goods. The worldwide spread left a window for a pandemic pressure of overstocking and buying. The threat of terror left many seeking for home resources, such as toilet paper, groceries, produce, sanitary wipes, hand sanitizers, bleach, and other home necessities as the public was frightened by the new outbreak. No one knew what was to be expected, only that every major store, such as Walmart, Target, and Costco, were left empty.

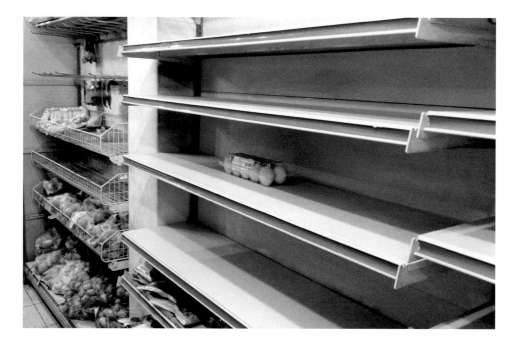

The out-of-stock items pushed the threat of COVID-19 and squeezed the issue of increasing panic more than ever. Popken (2020) stated,

Coronavirus has the potential to become a global pandemic, temporarily emptying retail store shelves in the coming months and depressing some consumer-facing businesses, experts say, with government officials advising families to take measured steps to stock up on certain essentials. A pandemic is the rapid spread of an infectious disease to a large amount of people in a short period of time across international boundaries.

With the shortage of food supplies and sanitation equipment, some could argue that the government has control of the virus; thus, meaning that this is an opportunity for global power of money and the growth of large business companies. However, with the spread of the virus, the outcome was more than gaining the power of money. The virus was more than an opportunity for corporations to make a few dollars. It was cutting off the livelihood and survival for the living and destroying humility without remorse.

As the virus changed the way of living, most businesses were to be the most impacted by the outbreak. As America shut down mainstream establishments, other countries followed. By the end of 2019, all major corporations, small businesses, social events, and active necessities for socioeconomic gatherings had been shut down.

3

EPIDEMIC SHUTDOWN

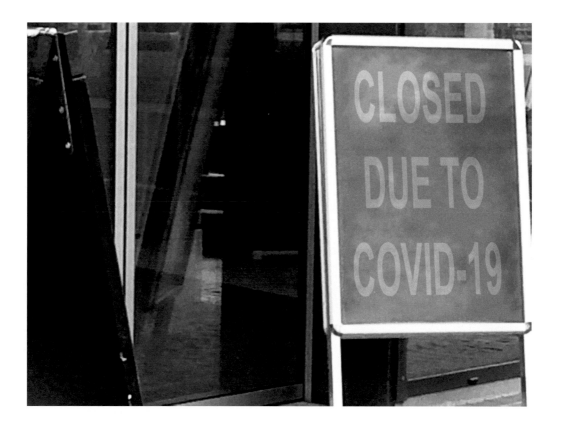

After the discovery of the virus, state officials, leaders, and presidents of world nations ordered a pandemic shutdown.

This was an order that ensured the safety or the spread of COVID-19. Creating an opportunity for the virus to spread was the key alternative by state and government officials. According to "A Timeline of COVID-19" (2020), on March 13, Trump declares COVID-19 a national emergency. President Donald Trump declares the novel coronavirus a national emergency and unlocks billions of dollars in federal funding to fight the disease's spread. On March 13, a travel ban on non-US citizens traveling from Europe went into effect; the Trump administration issues a travel ban on non-Americans who visited twenty-six European countries within fourteen days of coming to the United States. People traveling from the United Kingdom and the Republic of Ireland are exempted.

These were the first steps during the pandemic shutdown. Many felt that the shutdown was dramatic and needless. However, the virus was moving fast and infecting most of the world's population. The devastating outcome had been taking the lives of most elders, but with the non-social distancing in effect, the hopeful waited for the unexpected.

The virus shut down workers in every area, such as restaurants, bars and grills, schools, educational systems, city halls, government facilities, shopping establishments, and all places that included a gathering of five or more people.

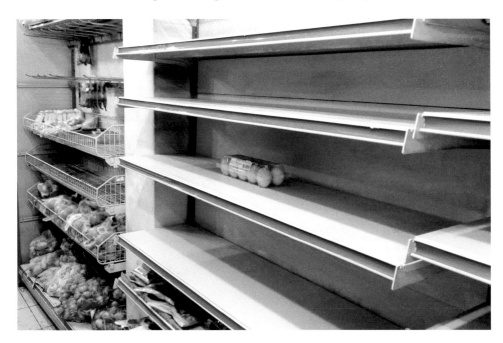

During the pandemic shutdown, many forgot how to live a fashion of living or conducting life without employment and or working. But most businesses that could stay open were establishments that provided commodities essential for living. Walmart was a key element that stayed open but was obligated to work under strict conditions and only operated during hours that are safe, not a twenty-four-hour workday.

According to Kochhar (2020):

> The COVID-19 outbreak and the economic downturn it engendered swelled the ranks of unemployed Americans by more than 14 million, from 6.2 million in February to 20.5 million in May 2020. As a result, the U.S. unemployment rate shot up from 3.8% in February – among the lowest on record in the post-World War II era – to 13.0% in May. That rate was the era's second highest, trailing only the level reached in April (14.4%).

The rise in the number of unemployed workers due to COVID-19 is substantially greater than the increase due to the Great Recession, when the number of unemployed increased by 8.8 million from the end of 2007 to the beginning of 2010. The Great Recession, which officially lasted from December 2007 to June 2009, pushed the unemployment rate to a peak of 10.6% in January 2010, considerably less than the rate currently, according to a new Pew Research Center analysis of government data.

The unemployment rate in May might have been as high as 16%, by the U.S. government's estimate. But it is not recorded as such because of measurement challenges that have arisen amid the coronavirus outbreak. Also, a sharp decline in labor force participation among U.S. workers overall may be adding to the understatement of unemployment. By May of 2019 9 million Americans in the labor force were out of a job compared to 5 million in February of 2019. But these workers are not included in the official measure of unemployment. Thus, the COVID-19 recession is comparable more to the Great Depression of the 1930s, when the unemployment rate is estimated to have reached 25%. Unemployment among all groups of workers increased sharply in the COVID-19 recession.

But the experiences of several groups of workers, such as women and black men, during the COVID-19 outbreak vary notably from how they experienced the Great Recession.

Here are five facts about how the COVID-19 downturn is affecting unemployment among American workers.

1. The unemployment rate for women in May (14.3%) was higher than the unemployment rate for men (11.9%).
2. The unemployment rate for black men in May (15.8%) was substantially less than the peak rate they faced in the Great Recession (21.2%).
3. Immigrants saw their unemployment rate jump higher than the rate for U.S.-born workers in the COVID-19 downturn, mirroring their experience in the Great Recession.
4. Workers in all but one age group saw their unemployment rate climb into the double digits in May due to the COVID-19 outbreak, unlike the Great Recession when this was true only for younger workers.
5. Unemployment rates in the COVID-19 downturn are lower among workers with higher levels of education, as in the Great Recession.

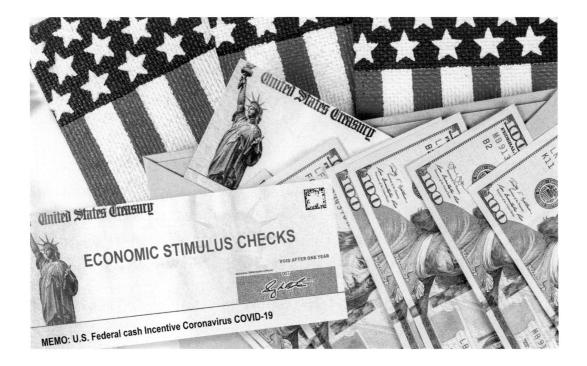

By March 2020, the world was in non-operational order, and most had been unemployed and or jobless. The virus was fighting in all areas and was stopping the production of how we lived and worked.

The global economic development of currency was on hold, but employment was rising with a disbursement of leaving many at home. The United States passed a three-trillion-dollar bill that would help Americans out with the problem of losing their jobs. The death toll increased as medical professionals strike to make progress for hospitalizing the ill.

With the virus in action, there was a stipulation about big corporations profiting from the pandemic. According to MacMillan (2020):

> year, collectively cutting more than 100,000 workers, *The Post* found. The data reveals a split screen inside many big companies this year. On one side, corporate leaders are touting their success and casting themselves as leaders on the road to economic recovery. On the other, many of their firms have put Americans out of work and used their profits to increase the wealth of shareholders.
>
> When the coronavirus struck, big companies promised to help battle the crisis. Dozens of prominent chief executives, who last year signed a public pledge to focus less on shareholders and more on the well-being of their employees and broader communities, appeared eager to make good on that promise. Many suspended payments to investors and vowed not to hold layoffs.

Then, 21 big firms that were profitable during the pandemic laid off workers anyway. Berkshire Hathaway raked in profits of $56 billion during the first six months of the pandemic while one of its subsidiary companies laid off more than 13,000 workers. Salesforce, Cisco Systems and PayPal cut staff even after their chief executives vowed not to do so.

Companies sent thousands of employees packing while sending billions of dollars to shareholders. Walmart, whose CEO spent the past year championing the idea that businesses "should not just serve shareholders," nonetheless distributed more than $10 billion to its investors during the pandemic while laying off 1,200 corporate office employees.

As the crisis rises the cost of living, transportation, food, medical treatment, cleaning supplies, and any other helpful necessities had been affected because of the threat of coronavirus.

Because of the shutdown and coronavirus moving fast among everyone, the fast-food industry was another sector set to profitably gain profit. The shutdown and contactless orders left all Americans seeking an appetite through delivery and or take out. According to Valinsky (2020):

McDonald's, Chipotle, Dunkin', Starbucks and several others reported earnings in recent weeks, which encompassed the brutal spring quarter when Covid-19 was rearing its head across the United States. In addition to illustrating how their bottom lines were decimated, the companies' quarterly financial updates also show how much we've changed our daily routines.

Here are five ways consumers' habits changed:

1. We're spending more and stocking up

Rather than coming in for coffee or a sandwich, we're buying lots more food in a single order. Starbucks (SBUX) said its average check size grew 25% in the most recent quarter because customers are purchasing multiple drinks and food items.

Dunkin (DNKN)' noticed a similar trend, with its average order amount growing because of "family-size bulk orders." Baskin-Robbins, which it also owns, said this partially offset a sales dip with more expensive orders because people are buying ice cream quarts and cakes. Stocking up also gave Domino's (DMPZF) a bump.

"One of the things that we have heard over the quarter is that customers are actively putting more food in the basket to have leftovers, the next day," CEO Ritch Allison said in a recent earnings call. "They're thinking about not just that evening's meal, but how they're planning for the following day."

2. Drive-thrus are thriving

The shift to a "contactless" experience was a boon for a lot of chains, including McDonald's (MCD). The company said roughly 90% of its US sales came through its drive-thru lanes and markets that have a lot of drive-thru locations are recovering faster.

Chipotle (CMG) has been aggressively expanding its drive-thrus and recently opened its 100th. Locations with Chipotlanes, as they are cleverly called, had 10% higher sales during the second quarter compared to company restaurants without them. Around 60% of its new locations planned this year will have drive-thrus.

Taco Bell-owner Yum! Brands (YUM) said it served an additional 5 million cars through its drive-thrus compared to the same time a year ago.

3. Digital sales are breaking records

Digital orders made through third-party services like Uber Eats or through chains' own apps also grew substantially in the quarter. Every company seems to have a digital success story, including McDonald's, Starbucks, Domino's, Chipotle, Yum! and Dunkin', all of which reported a spike in digital sales.

Chipotle's second-quarter digital sales grew a whopping 216% year-over-year and made up 61% of total sales. Yum! said digital orders at all of its brands (Taco Bell, Pizza Hut, and KFC) hit an all-time high, jumping $1 billion to $3.5 billion from the same quarter a year ago.

And Starbucks, which recently tweaked its app-based rewards program, said mobile orders encompassed 22% of all transactions, an increase of 6% compared to a year ago.

4. Breakfast is a bummer

The almost complete destruction of a morning commute for most of the country has had dire effects on the once-hot meal.

Coffee chains Dunkin' and Starbucks both reported deep declines in revenue and visits because people aren't stopping by as much in the mornings. Starbucks CEO Kevin Johnson CEO said the "disruption to the weekday morning routines, notably commuting to work and school, is a headwind."

Breakfast was previously a troublesome part of the day for McDonald's prior to Covid-19 and continues to be a drag on its sales. In addition to rising competition, the meal also "continues to be disproportionately impacted by disruptions to commuting routines," McDonald's CEO Chris Kempczinski said in this week's earnings call. Wendy's (WEN), which rolled out fancy new breakfast options just a few weeks before the pandemic, is set to release earnings next week.

5. Midday is the new morning

People might not be stopping in the early morning, but some are popping in a bit later. Starbucks said it's seeing spikes in traffic around 9:30 a.m. and again around 2 p.m., which has led the company to move employees' shifts toward those hours.

Dunkin' also noticed a similar trend, with sales shifting from early morning to midday between 11 am to 2 p.m. Those customers are buying non-coffee drinks, such as its new selection of teas, and snacks.

With fast food chains moving forward, they also had to consider the safety for customers and redesign their approach for serving customers. Therefore, all food industries had to follow federal guidelines when handling food for sale. All of these profit gains during the pandemic left small business closing their business and or falling into bankruptcy.

I like to give thanks to all those who worked in the food industry during the pandemic. They put in long hours and dedication to their art in the culinary industry.

4

SOCIAL DISTANCING AND REMEDIES

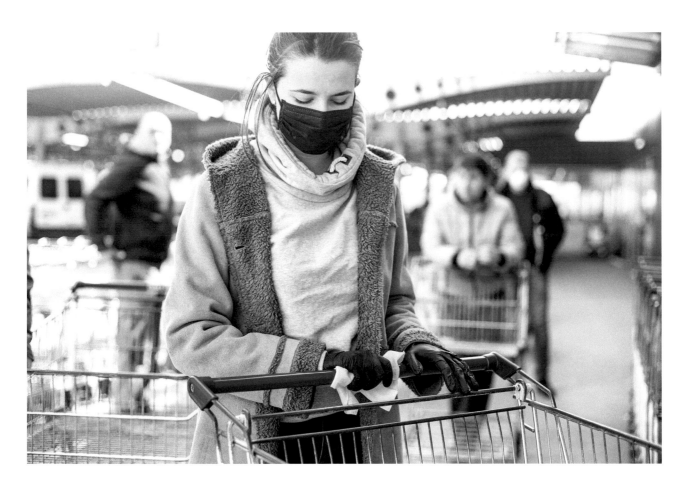

COVID-19 continues to weaken our lifestyle, economic system, and how we operate daily. The government implements new alternatives that will keep social gatherings to a minimum. The goal is to stop the spread of the virus by wearing a face mask and keeping six feet apart when outside. Social distancing is a must and has been deemed as a safety measure for others. But with educational systems on a downside, due to the virus social learning is a factor for many school institutions.

According to Maragakis (2020):

> The practice of social distancing means staying home and away from others as much as possible to help prevent the spread of COVID-19. The practice of social distancing encourages the use of things such as online video and phone communication instead of in-person contact.

> As communities reopen and people are more often in public, the term "physical distancing" (instead of social distancing) is being used to reinforce the need to stay at least 6 feet from others, as well as wearing face masks. Historically, social distancing was also used interchangeably to indicate physical distancing which is defined below. However, social distancing is a strategy distinct from physical distancing behavior. Wear a face mask or covering when you are not in your home and whenever you are around people who are not members of your household.

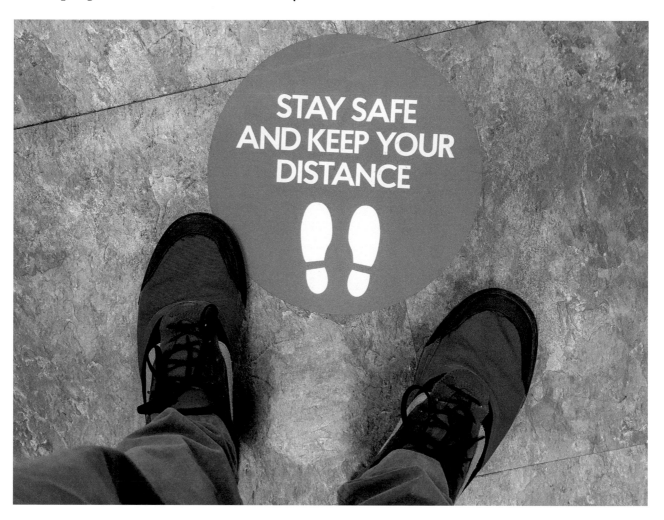

Maintain at least 6 feet of distance between yourself and others. Avoid crowded places, particularly indoors, and events that are likely to draw crowds. Other examples of social and physical distancing to avoid larger crowds or crowded spaces are:

- Working from home instead of at the office
- Closing schools or switching to online classes
- Visiting loved ones by electronic devices instead of in person
- Canceling or postponing conferences and large meetings

According to "COVID-19 Outbreak" (2022):

Scientists are still learning about COVID-19, the disease caused by the coronavirus, but according to the CDC, this highly contagious virus appears to be most commonly spread during close (within 6 feet) person-to-person contact through respiratory droplets.

"The means of transmission can be through respiratory droplets produced when a person coughs or sneezes, or by direct physical contact with an infected person, such as shaking hands," says Dr. David Goldberg, an internist and infectious disease specialist at NewYork-Presbyterian Medical Group Westchester and an assistant professor of medicine at Columbia University Vagelos College of Physicians and Surgeons.

The CDC also notes that COVID-19 can spread by airborne transmission, although this is less common than close contact with a person.

"Some infections can be spread by exposure to the virus in small droplets and particles that can linger in the air for minutes to hours," the CDC states. "These viruses may be able to infect people who are further than 6 feet away from the person who is infected or after that person has left the space. These transmissions occurred within enclosed spaces that had inadequate ventilation."

Finally, it's possible for coronavirus to spread through contaminated surfaces, but this is also less likely. According to the CDC, "Based on data from lab studies on COVID-19 and what we know about similar respiratory diseases, it may be possible that a person can get COVID-19 by touching a surface or object that has the virus on it and then touching their own mouth, nose, or possibly their eyes, but this isn't thought to be the main way the virus spreads."

Practice social distancing

Since close person-to-person contact appears to be the main source of transmission, social distancing remains a key way to mitigate spread. The CDC recommends maintaining a distance of approximately 6 feet from others in public places. This distance will help you avoid direct contact with respiratory droplets produced by coughing or sneezing.

In addition, studies have found that outdoor settings with enough space to distance and good ventilation will reduce the risk of exposure. "There is up to 80% less transmission of the virus happening outdoors versus indoors," says Dr. Ashwin Vasan, an assistant attending physician in the Department of Medicine at NewYork-Presbyterian/Columbia University Irving Medical Center and an assistant professor at the Mailman School of Public Health and Columbia University Vagelos College of Physicians and Surgeons.

"One study found that of 318 outbreaks that accounted for 1,245 confirmed cases in China, only one outbreak occurred outdoors. That's significant. I recommend spending time with others outside. We're not talking about going to a sporting event or a concert. We're talking about going for a walk or going to the park, or even having a conversation at a safe distance with someone outside."

Wash your hands

Practicing good hygiene is an important habit that helps prevent the spread of COVID-19. Make these CDC recommendations part of your routine:

- Wash your hands often with soap and water for at least 20 seconds, especially after you have been in a public place, or after blowing your nose, coughing, or sneezing.
- It's especially important to wash:

  ✓ Before eating or preparing food
  ✓ Before touching your face
  ✓ After using the restroom
  ✓ After leaving a public place

✓ After blowing your nose, coughing, or sneezing
✓ After handling your mask
✓ After changing a diaper
✓ After caring for someone who's sick
✓ After touching animals or pets

- If soap and water are not readily available, use a hand sanitizer that contains at least 60% alcohol. Cover all surfaces of your hands with the sanitizer and rub them together until they feel dry.
- Avoid touching your eyes, nose, and mouth with unwashed hands.

Visit the CDC website for guidelines on how to properly wash your hands and use hand sanitizer. And see our video below on how soap kills the coronavirus. There's plenty of science behind this basic habit. "Soap molecules disrupt the fatty layer or coat surrounding the virus," says Dr. Goldberg. "Once the viral coat is broken down, the virus is no longer able to function."

In addition to handwashing, disinfect frequently touched surfaces daily. This includes tables, doorknobs, light switches, countertops, handles, desks, phones, keyboards, toilets, faucets, and sinks.

Wear a mask

Face masks have become essential accessories in protecting yourself and others from contracting COVID-19.

The CDC recommends that people wear face coverings in public settings, especially since studies have shown that individuals with the novel coronavirus could be asymptomatic or presymptomatic. (Face masks, however, do not replace social distancing recommendations.)

"Face masks are designed to provide a barrier between your airway and the outside world," says Dr. Ole Vielemeyer, medical director of Weill Cornell ID Associates and Travel Medicine in the Division of Infectious Diseases at NewYork-Presbyterian/Weill Cornell Medical Center and Weill Cornell Medicine. "By wearing a mask that covers your mouth and nose, you will reduce the risk of serving as the source of disease spread by trapping your own droplets in the mask, and also reduce the risk of getting sick via droplets that contain the coronavirus by blocking access to your own airways."

Restrict your travel

Traveling can increase the spread of COVID-19 and put you at risk of contracting the disease. The CDC recommends avoiding non-essential travel to many international destinations during the pandemic. It also advises people to weigh the risks when it comes to domestic travel: "Travel increases your chance of getting and spreading COVID-19," states the CDC. "Staying home is the best way to protect yourself and others from COVID-19."

"For people at risk for the complications of COVID-19, such as those with underlying medical conditions or those who are older, it's prudent to avoid travel," says Dr. Goldberg.

If you must travel, take safety measures, consider your mode of transportation, and stay up to date on the restrictions that are in place at your destination. Adhering to your state's quarantine rules after traveling will help prevent the spread of COVID-19.

Watch for symptoms

The symptoms of infection for the coronavirus are often similar to those of other respiratory virus infections, such as influenza. Symptoms can include:

- ✓ Fever or chills
- ✓ Cough
- ✓ Shortness of breath or difficulty breathing
- ✓ Fatigue
- ✓ Muscle or body aches
- ✓ Headache
- ✓ New loss of taste or smell
- ✓ Sore throat
- ✓ Congestion or runny nose
- ✓ Nausea or vomiting
- ✓ Diarrhea

With the COVID-19 pandemic now coinciding with flu season, it's important to recognize the differences in symptoms—as well as get a flu shot. "The medical community is concerned that if we have an increased number of influenza cases, it will strain the hospital system on top of what's already going on with the COVID-19 pandemic," says Dr. Ting Wong, an attending physician and infectious disease specialist at New York-Presbyterian Brooklyn Methodist Hospital.

If you think you may have been exposed to a person with COVID-19 and have symptoms, call ahead to a doctor's office to see if you can get tested. All safety guidelines above can help.

Self-quarantine is a positive method that will provide safety and security for people that have COVID-19.

However, chloroquine phosphate, convalescent plasma therapy, Favipiravir, hydroxychloroquine, and remdesivir are just some of the drugs that are a trial for COVID-19, not a cure.

Chloroquine phosphate is a drug that is prescribed only in the United States. This is sold under the brand name Aralen and is distributed as tablets. This drug is prescribed to malaria patients and seems to be effective. According to "Chloroquine" (2020):

The clinical study information available at this time does not support the use of chloroquine for the treatment or prevention of COVID-19. Several chloroquine clinical studies were unable to find improvements in the treatment of COVID-19, such as to shorten hospital stay, to lessen the length or severity of the illness, or to reduce the number of deaths.

There also are concerns about side effects, such as an irregular heartbeat, and drug interactions that may occur from taking chloroquine.

Of note, the FDA approved an Emergency Use Authorization (EUA) on March 28, 2020, to allow chloroquine to treat adults and adolescents who weigh at least 110 pounds (50 kg) and who are hospitalized with COVID-19, but who are unable to participate in a clinical study. However, this recommendation was canceled on June 15, 2020, because clinical studies have not found that the use of chloroquine has shown substantial benefits for the treatment of COVID-19 compared to the risk of potential side effects.

Chloroquine should ONLY be taken under the direction of a doctor in a clinical study. Do not buy this medication online without a prescription.

If you experience irregular heartbeats, dizziness, or fainting while taking chloroquine, call 911 for emergency medical treatment. If you have other side effects, be sure to tell your doctor. Do not take chloroquine that is strictly intended for veterinary use – such as to treat fish in aquariums or for use in other animals – to treat or prevent COVID-19. The FDA reports that serious injury and death have been reported in people misusing these preparations.

Convalescent plasma is a recommended treatment but has little effect on the patients. This blood transfusion has helped some, but not many, COVID-19 victims. The process is not hard; however, it takes time for recovery. Because convalescent plasma is not yet approved by the Food Drug Administration, the health care providers should rely on data recovery for such administration on all COVID-19 patients.

Record keeping can help identify the progress of such trials. The focus is to ensure safety and accountability for underlining such possibilities for positive outcomes.

According to the Center for Biologics Evaluation and Research (2020):

On August 23, 2020, Food Drug Administration (FDA) issued an emergency use authorization (EUA) for COVID-19 convalescent plasma for the treatment of hospitalized patients with COVID-19. However, adequate and well-controlled randomized trials remain necessary for a definitive demonstration of COVID-19 convalescent plasma efficacy and to determine the optimal product attributes and appropriate patient populations for its use. Additional data will be forthcoming from other analyses and ongoing, well-controlled clinical trials. The ongoing clinical trials of investigational convalescent plasma should not be amended based on the issuance of the EUA; health care providers are encouraged to enroll patients in those trials.

Favipiravir is an antiviral drug; it's active in curing influenza and/or flu, a viral infection that attacks the respiratory system, the nose, throat, and lungs. It is commonly called the flu but is not the same as stomach flu. This progress has been slow and only clinical trials are provided. Japan is the cofounder of this drug, which was utilized to treat influenza. According to Marrow (2020):

A candidate drug for treating the new coronavirus, favipiravir, has produced promising results in early clinical trials in Russia. The clinical trial of 330 patients infected with the coronavirus should be finished by the end of May, said Andrei Ivashchenko, a professor at the Russian Academy of

Sciences and chairman of the board of directors at ChemRar, the company conducting the trials.

However, this drug was tested on animals before it has been administered to humans. This drug may have positive outcomes in low trials and could be the solution for overcoming this deadly virus. Medical trials are still being used during the ongoing pandemic.

Hydroxychloroquine is a drug that helps with the pain and swelling due to arthritis. This antirheumatic drug may prevent joint damage and reduce the high risk of disability. The Food Drug Administration has revoked the emergency use of such drugs due to the risk of heart rhythm problems. This drug is a family member of the medicines called "antimalaria," which also is classified as disease-modifying antirheumatic drug. This drug is most likely taken as a pill. Hydroxychloroquine is a drug that helps the treatment of malaria but is no longer used for such a purpose. However, after more research, the drug has been effective in treating lupus.

According to "Hydroxychloroquine" (2020):

> In 1956, the U.S. Food and Drug Administration approved Hydroxychloroquine for symptoms of lupus and rheumatoid arthritis, particularly skin inflammation, hair loss, mouth sores, fatigue, and joint pain.

> But like any other drug, there are some side effects. The use of Hydroxychloroquine has been known for visual change and or loss of vision. However, only those that use this drug at a high dose are at risk. It is recommended to have your eyes checked after one year of usage of the drug. According to Walker (2020) "The agency determined that the legal criteria for issuing an Emergency Use Authorization (EUA) are no longer met," according to Food Drug Administration (FDA) statement. Both hydroxychloroquine and a related antimalarial drug, chloroquine (CQ), are "unlikely to be effective at treating COVID-19" for uses described in the EUA.

> Moreover, the FDA now says the benefits of the drug "no longer outweigh the potential risks," citing the serious cardiac adverse events associated with the drug. "This warrants revocation of the EUA for HCQ and CQ for the treatment of COVID-19," the agency said.

However, while current FDA guidelines did not recommend the use of the drugs outside of a randomized clinical trial, the FDA also pointed to recent data from a large clinical trial showing no "evidence of benefit" for mortality, effect on hospital length of stay, or need for mechanical ventilation among COVID-19 patients treated with hydroxychloroquine.

Finally, the last drug that is at the top of the list is remdesivir, which does not give a solution to the ongoing pandemic. Like any other drug, it is unstable for COVID-19 patients' use. This injection helps the spread of the virus throughout the body and is given once a day for five to ten days. According to Schmidt (2020):

> Remdesivir is an antiviral medication originally developed by biopharmaceutical company Gilead Sciences to treat Ebola. Although the drug didn't work well against that disease, it later showed promise fighting Severe Acute Respiratory Syndrome (SARS) and Middle East Respiratory (MERS) illnesses caused by coronaviruses in animal studies, which is why researchers thought remdesivir might help fight COVID-19. Remdesivir is designed to slow or stop the virus from creating copies of itself by blocking this particular enzyme.

> The drug works differently than antibody-based treatments or vaccines, which are designed to help a person's immune system identify and eliminate pathogens. Remdesivir is most effective when given early as soon as patients begin to show symptoms. But giving the drug early in an infection is a challenge because it is administered to the patient over 10 days. While the remdesivir development is an important first step, is still a long way from FDA-approved therapies that are proven to prevent or treat COVID-19. The first antibody-based treatments could become available in the year 2020 and will help the process for recovery of COVID-19.

5

BLACK LIVES MATTER

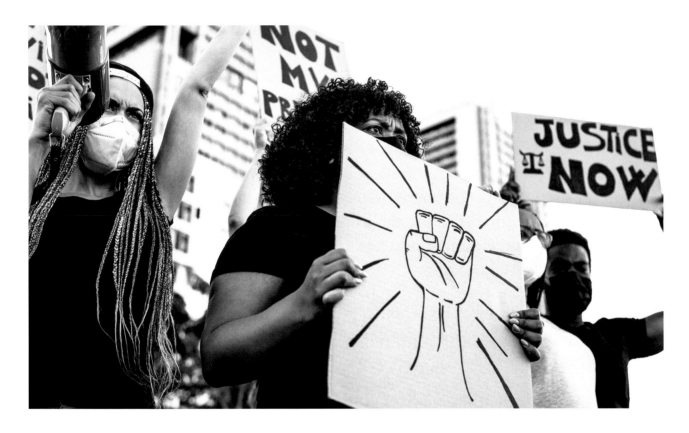

As the virus counts down and kills many, there is another fight for other reasons that enable social distancing. George Floyd was the victim of a wrongful police arrest and started a movement that highlighted outrage against the pandemic. As many around the world were shocked that the virus had been moving fast, the world was fastened by the deadly outcome of George Floyd.

According to Hill (2020):

> On May 25, Minneapolis police officers arrested George Floyd, a 46-year-old black man, after a convenience store employee called 911 and told the police that Mr. Floyd had bought cigarettes with a counterfeit $20 bill. Seventeen minutes after the first squad car arrived at the scene, Mr. Floyd was unconscious and pinned beneath three police officers, showing no signs of life.

It was said that the pinning of Mr. Floyd to the ground for at least eight minutes and fifteen seconds was all it took to kill a man that was no threat to others around him.

Many marched in the name of defense against racial threats of hate by the Minneapolis police officers. However, the launch for a new fight was counting down and revealed the anger among Americans and nations around the world. As the cases of coronavirus increase, the protest for George Floyd rises with a strong voice. The battle of a new alarming surge peeked throughout the world and people unit to help the unjust death of a helpless man. While the media creates a motivation for some to help with the rioting among business owners, public officials, police officers, and noncolored people, some are outraged by the wrongful outcome of what was supposed to be a promising year, 2020.

This led to protests that shook the world and left many questioning how officers practiced the law in the community. According to "Black Lives Matter DC v. Trump" (2022):

> On June 1, 2020, Black Lives Matter protesters gathered in Lafayette Square Park near the White House to protest against police brutality and the police killing of George Floyd and Breonna Taylor.
>
> In a violation of civil rights and what the *New York Times* named "one of the defining moments of the Trump presidency," then President Trump and his administration called upon law enforcement to use force and violence to remove protesters from the area, without warning. A short while later, President Trump walked across the street to a nearby church St Johns for a photo op.
>
> Protesters were hurt, media personnel were attacked, and church volunteers and clergy were pushed off the patio of St. Johns and tear-gassed. In response, the ACLU of DC filed to sue President Trump, Attorney General Barr, Secretary of Defense Esper, the D.C. Metropolitan Police department and

numerous other federal officials on behalf of Black Lives Matter D.C. and other plaintiffs affected.

And while what happened on June 1st shocked many of us, for civil rights activists it was a very familiar story, something to add to a long list of similar incidents. Freedom of speech and assembly are important tools in the fight for civil rights, but these rights, when exercised by Black Americans, are frequently met with violent pushback from authorities.

The year 2020 is a turnaround year to make things right and/or be the year for seeking new dreams or big goals. But it will be the year known for civil rights for all color and/or those who have been victims of bad policing.

6

CONCLUSIONS

In conclusion, the real identity of humanity has been changed. The deadly outbreak has had all nations collaborating for the act of doing good. With every nation falling to the end of a new discovery, we have united for individualism and peace because of this impact. However, some will argue that this was not manipulated and/or controlled. I thank all of them that helped during the pandemic and helped in the process of stopping the spread of the virus.

And for those who passed on and/or were affected by the virus, I give my condolences and deepest prayer. I hope that all this information has helped to process such a bad outcome in life. The main objective of this project is to help those who knew little about the coronavirus and give details about the year 2020.

REFERENCES

"A Timeline of COVID-19 Developments in 2020." 2020. Retrieved September 02, 2020. https://www.ajmc.com/view/a-timeline-of-covid19-developments-in-2020.

"About COVID-19." 2020. Retrieved August 30, 2020. https://www.cdc.gov/coronavirus/2019-ncov/cdcresponse/about-COVID-19.html.

American Civil Liberties Union. 2022. "Black lives matter DC v. Trump." Retrieved August 15, 2022. https://www.aclu.org/podcast/black-lives-matter-dc-v-trump.

Center for Biologics Evaluation and Research. "Investigational COVID-19 Convalescent Plasma - Emergency INDs." 2020. Retrieved September 28, 2020. https://www.fda.gov/vaccines-blood-biologics/investigational-new-drug-ind-or-device-exemption-ide-process-cber/recommendations-investigational-covid-19-convalescent-plasma.

Center for Disease Control and Prevention. 2020. "Public Health Guidance for Potential COVID-19 Exposure Associated with International or Domestic Travel." Retrieved September 14, 2020. https://www.cdc.gov/coronavirus/2019-ncov/php/risk-assessment.html.

"Chloroquine (Oral Route) Side Effects." 2020. Retrieved September 14, 2020. https://www.mayoclinic.org/drugs-supplements/chloroquine-oral-route/side-effects/drg-20062834?p=1.

Cohut, Maria. 2020. "What is the global impact of the new coronavirus pandemic?" *Medical News Today*, January 16. Retrieved August 30, 2020. https://www.medicalnewstoday.com/articles/covid-19-global-impact-how-the-coronavirus-is-affecting-the-world.

"Coronavirus COVID-19 Definitions, Abbreviations, Acronyms, Full Forms." n.d. Retrieved August 26, 2020. https://relief.unboundmedicine.com/relief/view/Coronavirus-Guidelines/2355004/all/Coronavirus_Glossary_of_Terms.

"COVID-19 situation update worldwide, as of 11 September 2020." 2020. Retrieved September 14, 2020. https://www.ecdc.europa.eu/en/geographical-distribution-2019-ncov-cases.

Dictionary. (n.d.). Retrieved September 02, 2020, from https://www.dictionary.com/browse/virus?s=t

Hill, E. et al. 2020. "How George Floyd Was Killed in Police Custody." *New York Times*, June 1. Retrieved October 15, 2020, from https://www.nytimes.com/2020/05/31/us/george-floyd-investigation.html.

"Hydroxychloroquine: Benefits, Side Effects, and Dosing." n.d. Retrieved September 28, 2020. https://www.lupus.org/resources/drug-spotlight-on-hydroxychloroquine.

Kochhar, Rakesh. 2020. "Unemployment rose higher in three months of COVID-19 than it did in two years of the Great Recession." Pew Research. Retrieved September 13, 2020. https://www.pewresearch.org/fact-tank/2020/06/11/unemployment-rose-higher-in-three-months-of-covid-19-than-it-did-in-two-years-of-the-great-recession/.

MacMillan, Douglas J. 2020. "America's biggest companies are flourishing during the pandemic and putting thousands of people out of work." *The Washington Post*, December 16. Retrieved August 15, 2022. https://www.washingtonpost.com/graphics/2020/business/50-biggest-companies-coronavirus-layoffs/.

Maragakis, Lisa L. 2020. "Coronavirus, Social and Physical Distancing and Self-Quarantine." John Hopkins Medicine. Retrieved September 14, 2020. https://www.hopkinsmedicine.org/health/conditions-and-diseases/coronavirus/coronavirus-social-distancing-and-self-quarantine.

Marrow, A. 2020. "Russia's ChemRar says in second-, third-phase testing of coronavirus drug favipiravir." Reuters, May 14. Retrieved September 28, 2020. https://www.reuters.com/article/us-health-coronavirus-russia-drug/russias-chemrar-says-in-second-third-phase-testing-of-coronavirus-drug-favipiravir-idUSKBN22Q2SW.

MedlinePlus. "Chloroquine." n.d. MedlinePlus. Retrieved September 14, 2020. https://medlineplus.gov/druginfo/meds/a682318.html.

NewYork-Presbyterian. 2022. "Coronavirus Prevention: How to Protect Yourself from COVID-19." Health Matters. Retrieved August 15, 2022. https://healthmatters.nyp.org/how-to-protect-yourself-from-coronavirus-covid-19/.

Popken, B. 2020. "Coronavirus epidemic: U.S. retailers could see some empty shelves by mid-April." NBC News, February 28. Retrieved August 31, 2020. https://www.nbcnews.com/business/consumer/u-s-could-see-some-empty-shelves-mid-april-if-n1144351.

Sandhu, V. 2020. "Hydroxychloroquine (Plaquenil)." American College of Rheumatology. Retrieved September 28, 2020. https://www.rheumatology.org/I-Am-A/Patient-Caregiver/Treatments/Hydroxychloroquine-Plaquenil.

Schmidt, M. 2020. "What Is Remdesivir, the First Drug That Treats Coronavirus?" Retrieved September 28, 2020. https://www.discovermagazine.com/health/what-is-remdesivir-the-first-drug-that-treats-coronavirus.

Stock images, photos, vectors, video, and music. Shutterstock. (n.d.). Retrieved August 16, 2022, from https://www.shutterstock.com/.

Valinsky, J. 2020. "5 ways the coronavirus changed how we Eat Fast Food." CNN, August 1. Retrieved August 16, 2022. https://www.cnn.com/2020/08/01/business/fast-food-coronavirus-habits/index.html.

Walker, Molly. 2020. "HCQ No Longer Approved Even a Little for COVID-19." *MedPage Today*, June 15. Retrieved September 28, 2020. https://www.medpagetoday.com/infectiousdisease/covid19/87066.

Williams, S. 2020. *The Scientist.*

Printed in the United States
by Baker & Taylor Publisher Services